HASHIMOTO'S THYROIDITIS

MEANS OF PREVENTING ALL THE CAUSES OF HASHIMOTO'S THYROIDITIS

DR. A. RAMOS

Contents

INTRODUCTION

An autoimmune condition called Hashimoto's Thyroiditis affects the thyroid gland, a little gland at the front of the neck that resembles a butterfly. Hashimoto's Thyroiditis, named for the Japanese physician Dr. Hakaru Hashimoto, who initially reported the ailment in 1912, is the most frequent cause of hypothyroidism, or an underactive thyroid, in many regions of the world.

The immune system incorrectly perceives the thyroid gland as a threat in Hashimoto's thyroiditis, leading to the production of antibodies that target and harm the gland. Thyroid tissue gradually deteriorates as a result of this immune reaction, making it more difficult for the thyroid to generate thyroid hormones. These hormones play a critical role in controlling the body's metabolism, which includes producing energy and controlling body temperature.

Women are more likely to get Hashimoto's thyroiditis, and the condition frequently develops gradually. In the early stages of the illness, many people may not exhibit any symptoms at all. But hypothyroidism can cause symptoms including weariness, weight gain, cold intolerance, dry skin, and mood swings as thyroid function deteriorates.

Blood tests are commonly used in diagnosis to check for the presence of particular antibodies linked to autoimmune thyroid diseases and to evaluate thyroid hormone levels. Hormone replacement therapy, which uses synthetic thyroid hormones to address the underactive thyroid function, is a common treatment for Hashimoto's thyroiditis.

Since untreated hypothyroidism can result in a number of issues, it's critical for people with Hashimoto's thyroiditis to collaborate closely with medical professionals in order to manage their illness. To maintain healthy thyroid hormone levels and reduce symptoms, further monitoring and medication modifications could be required.

Recognizing the autoimmune nature of Hashimoto's thyroiditis, its effects on thyroid function, and the significance of early detection and treatment are all necessary to comprehend the condition. Hashimoto's is an autoimmune disease that emphasizes the intricate interactions between the immune system and the body's own tissues, highlighting the necessity for all-encompassing and customized treatment plans.

CHAPTER ONE

An explanation of Hashimoto's thyroiditis

Named for the 1912 description of the autoimmune condition Hashimoto's Thyroiditis by the Japanese physician Dr. Hakaru Hashimoto, it is characterized by persistent inflammation of the thyroid gland. The thyroid gland, which is situated near the front of the neck, produces thyroid hormones such triiodothyronine (T3) and thyroxine (T4), which are essential for controlling metabolism.

When thyroid tissue is misidentified as foreign by the immune system, an immune reaction is triggered against it, resulting in Hashimoto's thyroiditis. Thyroid hormone synthesis declines as a result of inflammation and the immune attack's progressive elimination of thyroid cells. Because of this, people who have Hashimoto's thyroiditis frequently experience hypothyroidism, a disorder in which the thyroid gland is underactive.

Nature of Autoimmune:

As an autoimmune condition, Hashimoto's thyroiditis occurs when the immune system of the body, which is meant to defend against external invaders, accidentally targets one of its own tissues, in this case, the thyroid gland.

Slow Onset:

Hashimoto's thyroiditis usually develops gradually, and it may not show any symptoms in the early stages. Hypothyroidism is brought on by inflammation and thyroid tissue destruction as the autoimmune disease worsens.

Occurrence:

One of the most frequent causes of hypothyroidism is Hashimoto's thyroiditis, which primarily affects women while it can also strike men. It can appear at any time in life, but it usually does so in middle age.

Signs of hypothyroidism include:

People with Hashimoto's thyroiditis may exhibit hypothyroidism symptoms as their thyroid function deteriorates. These may manifest as weariness, weight gain, cold sensitivity, dry skin, hair loss, and mood swings.

Blood tests are used in the diagnosis process to determine thyroid hormone (T4, T3) and thyroid-stimulating hormone (TSH) levels. It is frequently possible to detect the presence of certain antibodies, such as anti-thyroid peroxidase (TPO) antibodies, which confirms the autoimmune origin of the illness.

Therapy:

Levothyroxine, a synthetic thyroid hormone, is commonly used in hormone replacement therapy for Hashimoto's thyroiditis in order to compensate for the underactive thyroid. To maintain appropriate thyroid hormone levels, prescription modifications and routine monitoring are common.

Problems:

If untreated, goiter (enlargement of the thyroid gland) and, in rare instances, thyroid nodules or thyroid cancer can occur as a result of Hashimoto's thyroiditis.

Handling Hashimoto's Thyroiditis necessitates a multifaceted strategy that takes into account the autoimmune component of the illness as well as the correlated hypothyroidism. For those with Hashimoto's thyroiditis, collaborating closely with medical professionals such as endocrinologists helps them reach optimal thyroid function and enhances their general health.

Reasons and the Nature of Autoimmune Disease

Because Hashimoto's thyroiditis is autoimmune in origin, the thyroid gland is wrongly targeted and attacked by the immune system. Although the precise causes of autoimmune diseases such as Hashimoto's thyroiditis remain unclear, a confluence of hormonal, environmental, and genetic variables is thought to be involved.

Genetic Elements:

Hashimoto's thyroiditis is one of the autoimmune thyroid diseases that has a strong genetic propensity. Hashimoto's disease may be more common in people with a family history of autoimmune diseases, particularly thyroid conditions.

Environmental Stressors:

Hashimoto's thyroiditis is believed to be triggered by a variety of environmental variables, especially in genetically predisposed individuals. These triggers could include food factors, stress, exposure to specific chemicals, or diseases.

Infections

Infections caused by bacteria or viruses can set off the onset of autoimmune disorders. It is thought that infections can trigger an immunological reaction that could cause the immune system to mistakenly target the thyroid gland in those who are susceptible.

Hormonal Elements:

Endocrine shifts, such those brought on by puberty, pregnancy, or menopause, might affect how autoimmune thyroid diseases manifest or worsen. Alterations in the equilibrium of hormones can affect the control of the immune system and lead to autoimmune reactions.

Immune System Impairment:

When someone has Hashimoto's thyroiditis, their immune system misinterprets thyroid tissue as foreign material rather than seeing it as a component of their body. Antibodies are produced in response, particularly anti-thyroglobulin and anti-thyroid peroxidase (TPO) antibodies, which target and harm thyroid cells.

T cells' function:

T cells, or T lymphocytes, are important players in the autoimmune process. T cells that have invaded the thyroid gland and released cytokines signaling molecules that promote inflammation and an increased immune response are the cause of Hashimoto's thyroiditis.

Damage Mediated by Antibodies:

One of the main characteristics of Hashimoto's thyroiditis is the presence of antibodies, namely anti-TPO antibodies. Thyroid function is hampered, thyroid cell death occurs, and inflammation is caused by these antibodies that target enzymes involved in the synthesis of thyroid hormone.

Development of Hypothyroidism:

As the thyroid's capacity to generate enough thyroid hormones declines over time, the autoimmune attack on the gland may cause hypothyroidism. Thyroid function declines as a result of the slow death of thyroid tissue.

Recognizing the intricate interactions between immune system malfunction, environmental triggers, and hereditary susceptibility is necessary to comprehend the autoimmune nature of Hashimoto's thyroiditis. The ultimate consequence is the generation of antibodies that target the thyroid gland, causing inflammation, damage, and the onset of hypothyroidism, even though the precise triggers may differ from person to person. The goal of ongoing study is to learn more about the triggers and development of autoimmune thyroid diseases.

Signs and Gradual Incidence

The symptoms of Hashimoto's thyroiditis may not appear right away and frequently develop gradually. The degree of symptoms may escalate with time as the autoimmune reaction against the thyroid gland persists, and the condition's course can differ from person to person. The following are typical signs of Hashimoto's thyroiditis:

Weary:

Common symptoms include an overall sense of exhaustion and persistent weariness. Even after receiving enough sleep, some people may feel lethargic.

Gain of Weight:

Unexpected weight gain is a typical indicator of hypothyroidism linked to Hashimoto's thyroiditis, even in the absence of considerable dietary or exercise modifications.

Sensitivity to Cold:

Feelings of persistent coldness may result from an increase in sensitivity to low temperatures. Common signs include cold hands and feet.

Dry Hair and Skin:

Hypothyroidism is characterized by brittle and dry hair, as well as dry, rough, and pale skin. There may be significant changes to the skin's and hair's texture and appearance.

Constipation:

Constipation and slow bowel movements are typical signs of hypothyroidism. Reduced thyroid hormone production might cause the digestive system to slow down.

Muscle Pain and Weakness:

It is possible to experience muscle weakness, pains, and stiffness, which makes physical activity more difficult. There may also be muscle cramping and joint discomfort.

Changes in Mood and Depression:

Hypothyroidism may be linked to mood swings, such as depressive symptoms, impatience, and trouble concentrating.

irregularities in menstruation:

Changes in the menstrual cycle, such as heavier or irregular menstrual flow, irregular periods, or more discomfort during the menstrual process, might affect women who have Hashimoto's thyroiditis.

Hair Loss:

There may be hair loss and thinning, especially from the scalp. Hair texture changes and increased fragility are frequent occurrences.

CHAPTER TWO

Goiter, or swelling of the neck:

There are situations when an enlarged thyroid gland causes an obvious swelling in the front of the neck. A goiter is what this is called, and it might or might not hurt.

Deficit in Computational Ability:

Cognitive dysfunction brought on by hypothyroidism can result in memory loss, concentration issues, and an overall sense of mental fog.

It's crucial to remember that not everyone with Hashimoto's thyroiditis will have all of these symptoms, and some may be mild or caused by unrelated conditions. Furthermore, there might be variations in the course of the illness, and some people may experience intervals of symptom remission interspersed with flare-ups.

Individuals should seek medical assistance for accurate diagnosis and management if they suspect they have Hashimoto's Thyroiditis or if their symptoms are chronic. Tests on blood that measure antibodies and thyroid hormone levels can assist determine the proper course of treatment and establish the existence of an autoimmune disease.

Blood tests, imaging scans, and medical evaluations are used in the diagnosis of Hashimoto's thyroiditis. Thyroid function is evaluated, certain antibodies are looked for, and other possible reasons of thyroid dysfunction are ruled out. The following are important facets of Hashimoto's thyroiditis diagnosis and medical evaluation:

Clinical Evaluation:

A comprehensive clinical examination involving a review of the patient's medical history, symptoms, and risk factors will be performed by a healthcare professional. It may be especially important to know about any family history of autoimmune thyroid problems.

Physical Assessment:

To evaluate the size, texture, and presence of any enlargement (goiter) in the thyroid gland, a physical examination may be conducted. Other physical symptoms including dry skin, changes in hair, and swelling might also be checked for by the healthcare professional.

Blood Examinations:

In order to diagnose Hashimoto's thyroiditis, blood tests are essential. The blood tests listed below are frequently performed:

Thyroid Hormone Levels (TSH, Free T4, Free T3): Thyroid function is evaluated by measuring the levels of thyroid hormones (T4 and T3) and thyroid-stimulating hormone (TSH).

Thyroid Antibody Tests: These consist of anti-thyroglobulin and anti-thyroid peroxidase (TPO) antibodies. Increased concentrations of these antibodies signify thyroid gland-specific autoimmune activity.

Imaging with ultrasound:

The thyroid gland may occasionally undergo an ultrasonography to see its size, composition, and any anomalies. This imaging study can be used to determine whether nodules or a goiter are present.

Biopsy with Fine Needle Aspiration (FNA):

To rule out thyroid cancer, a fine needle aspiration biopsy may be suggested if thyroid nodules are found during imaging. This entails removing a tiny sample of the nodule's tissue for analysis.

Eliminate Extra Causes:

The goal of the medical evaluation is to rule out any other possible reasons of thyroid dysfunction, including bacterial or viral infections, side effects from medication, and other autoimmune conditions.

Advice from an Endocrinologist:

For additional assessment and treatment in certain circumstances, speaking with an endocrinologist a specialist in problems connected to hormones may be advised.

Monitoring and Follow-Up:

In order to evaluate thyroid function and modify treatment as appropriate, ongoing monitoring is frequently required. Repeat blood tests to monitor antibodies and thyroid hormone levels may be part of routine follow-up sessions.

The procedure of diagnosing Hashimoto's thyroiditis involves cooperation between patients and medical professionals. Accurate diagnosis of Hashimoto's disease requires additional assessment and confirmation by antibody testing if the condition is suspected based on symptoms or preliminary blood tests. In order to address the autoimmune process, relieve symptoms, and avoid consequences related to hypothyroidism, early detection and effective management are essential. People who are at risk for thyroid issues or who are exhibiting symptoms should consult a doctor for a thorough assessment.

Methods of Therapy

Treating Hashimoto's thyroiditis primarily aims to control the inflammatory reaction, lessen inflammation, and treat the ensuing hypothyroidism with synthetic thyroid hormones. The following are the primary methods of treating Hashimoto's thyroiditis:

Therapy Using Thyroid Hormone Replacement:

Thyroid hormone replacement treatment is the mainstay of care for patients with Hashimoto's thyroiditis. Levothyroxine, a synthetic version of the thyroid hormone thyroxine, is the most often prescribed drug (T4). Levothyroxine aids in the body's return to normal thyroid hormone levels.

Customized Dosage Modifications:

Individualized thyroid hormone replacement therapy dosages are determined by considerations like age, weight, symptoms, and the degree of hypothyroidism. It is essential to regularly check thyroid hormone levels through blood tests in order to modify the dosage of medicine as necessary.

Adherence to Medication Consistently:

People with Hashimoto's thyroiditis must take their thyroid hormone replacement therapy on a regular basis and according to their doctor's instructions. Adjusting thyroid hormone levels and managing symptoms may be impacted by missing or deviating from the recommended dosage.

Observation and Succession:

It's crucial to schedule follow-up visits with medical professionals in order to check thyroid function via blood testing. These findings may warrant modifying the dosage of the medicine.

Handling Symptom Management:

While the underlying hypothyroidism is treated with thyroid hormone replacement, some symptoms of Hashimoto's thyroiditis, like weariness and dry skin, may not go away. Supportive actions, such upholding a healthy lifestyle and controlling stress, can assist in reducing these symptoms.

Handling Goiter:

When a goiter, or enlarged thyroid gland, is present, treatment options may include managing the underlying inflammation and, in certain situations, thinking about procedures like medication or surgery.

Antioxidant and Inflammatory Interventions:

Some people might look into dietary and lifestyle changes that promote general health and may reduce inflammation. In addition to medical care, antioxidant-rich diets, consistent exercise, and stress-reduction strategies may be taken into consideration.

Handling Concurrent Conditions:

Adrenal insufficiency or celiac disease are examples of concomitant illnesses that may affect people with Hashimoto's thyroiditis. When these problems are present, managing them is essential to the entire course of treatment.

It is noteworthy that although replacement of thyroid hormones effectively addresses the hypothyroidism linked to Hashimoto's disease, the autoimmune aspect of the ailment remains unabated. To maintain normal thyroid function and general health, continuous monitoring and control are required as the underlying immunological reaction may endure.

Patients with Hashimoto's thyroiditis should collaborate closely with endocrinologists and other medical professionals to create a personalized treatment plan that is effective and meets their needs. To effectively manage Hashimoto's thyroiditis and optimize thyroid health, open communication, routine follow-up, and adherence to prescribed medications are essential.

Lifestyle Factors to Take Into Account

Aside from pharmaceutical interventions, lifestyle choices can be crucial in controlling Hashimoto's thyroiditis and promoting general health. For those with Hashimoto's thyroiditis, the following lifestyle aspects should be taken into account:

A balanced, nutrient-rich diet can promote general health. A range of fruits, vegetables, whole grains, lean proteins, and healthy fats should be included. Some people with Hashimoto's thyroiditis might look into anti-inflammatory or Mediterranean diets, as they may be beneficial in reducing inflammation.

Sensitivity to gluten:

A small percentage of people with Hashimoto's thyroiditis may also have celiac disease or gluten intolerance. If removing gluten improves your symptoms or antibody levels, you might want to think about switching to a gluten-free diet. However, before making big dietary changes, it's imperative to speak with a doctor or a qualified dietician.

Frequent Workout:

Frequent exercise supports metabolism, aids in stress management, and enhances general wellbeing. Pick enjoyable activities like yoga, swimming, or walking, and try to incorporate both strength- and aerobic-training activities into your routine.

Handling Stress:

Prolonged stress might affect thyroid function and make Hashimoto's thyroiditis symptoms worse. Use stress-reduction strategies including mindfulness, deep breathing, meditation, and other relaxation exercises. Getting enough sleep is also essential for stress management and maintaining general wellness.

Sufficient Sleep:

Make sure you get enough good sleep every night. Set up a regular sleep schedule and aim for 7-9 hours of sleep each night. Thyroid hormone control, like other hormone regulatory processes, depends on sleep.

Reducing Toxins in the Environment:

Certain people might be more vulnerable to poisons in the environment. Reduce your exposure to substances that may cause thyroid disruption, such as pesticides, plastics, and other chemicals present in household goods.

Frequent Observation:

Make an effort to take charge of your health by scheduling routine check-ups and having blood tests done to check thyroid function. Check-ups with healthcare professionals on a regular basis help guarantee that treatment plans are in line with your health objectives and that medication dosages are acceptable.

Complementary Medicines:

Think about complementary therapies that could improve general health. With the advice and consent of medical professionals, one may investigate acupuncture, massage, and other complementary or alternative therapies.

Compliance with Medication:

Follow the instructions for taking the thyroid hormone replacement drug as directed. For stable thyroid hormone levels, make sure you take your medicine as prescribed by your doctor.

Resources for Education:

Learn about autoimmune diseases and Hashimoto's thyroiditis. Recognize the ailment, available treatments, and lifestyle implications. Reputable websites, support groups, and educational resources can offer insightful knowledge and a feeling of connection.

It's important to remember that lifestyle factors should be examined with medical professionals to make sure they complement unique demands and objectives for health. Since every patient with Hashimoto's thyroiditis is different, successful management requires a tailored strategy that includes working with medical specialists.

Psychological Wellness

One of the most important aspects of general health is emotional well-being, which has a big influence on people with Hashimoto's thyroiditis. Stress management, symptom management, and cultivating an optimistic outlook are all important components in managing the emotional aspects of having a chronic illness.

CHAPTER THREE

When treating Hashimoto's thyroiditis, keep the following in mind for your emotional health:

Honest Communication

Encourage candid dialogue with medical professionals. Together with your medical team, discuss your worries, inquiries, and personal experiences as you attempt to manage the psychological as well as the physical symptoms of Hashimoto's thyroiditis.

Knowledge and Self-determination:

Learn about the signs and treatments of Hashimoto's thyroiditis. Education enables people to take an active role in their care and gain a better understanding of their disease.

Assist Mechanism:

Create a network of friends and relatives, as well as any other people who may be affected by Hashimoto's thyroiditis. Emotional well-being can be enhanced by receiving empathy, sharing experiences, and surrounding oneself with supportive people.

Body-Mind Techniques:

Include mind-body exercises in your program, such yoga, mindfulness, or meditation. These techniques can lessen tension, promote calmness, and strengthen emotional fortitude.

Writing a Journal:

To keep note of your feelings, symptoms, and any trends you notice, think about starting a journal. Keeping a journal can help you understand how physical problems and mental health are related.

Creating Reasonable Objectives:

Make sure your goals are attainable and reasonable. Divide more difficult jobs into smaller, more doable segments, and acknowledge your progress as you go. This strategy can lessen overwhelming feelings.

Expression of Emotions:

Permit yourself to feel what you're feeling. Whether it's through writing, drawing, or conversing with a buddy, expressing your emotions can be healing.

Seek Expert Assistance:

If necessary, think about getting help from a mental health specialist. Help with stress management, emotional processing, and creating plans to preserve emotional health can be obtained from a therapist or counselor.

Positivity in Thought:

Develop an optimistic outlook by emphasizing the things in life that make you happy and grateful. Recognize the difficulties associated with living with a chronic illness and treat yourself with kindness and self-compassion.

Self-Healing Techniques:

Make self-care activities that support emotional health a priority. These include getting enough sleep, doing things you like, and setting aside time for relaxation.

Adaptation and Acceptance:

Recognize and understand that managing your Hashimoto's thyroiditis may need you to adjust to new situations. Accept adaptability and resiliency when handling any obstacles that may come up.

Honor minor victories:

Acknowledge and celebrate minor victories in your health management. Acknowledging accomplishment can improve morale, whether it's taking medication consistently, forming better behaviors, or accomplishing personal goals.

Recall that maintaining emotional well-being is a continuous endeavor, and that dealing with a chronic illness is natural to cause a range of feelings. You can cultivate emotional resilience and lay a solid foundation for effectively managing Hashimoto's thyroiditis by incorporating these factors into your daily routine.

Possible Difficulties and Surveillance

If Hashimoto's thyroiditis is not treated or is not managed well, it can cause a number of problems. To identify changes in thyroid function and quickly address any potential issues, routine monitoring is crucial. The following are possible side effects and methods for keeping an eye on Hashimoto's thyroiditis:

Insufficient thyroid function

The main side effect of Hashimoto's thyroiditis is hypothyroidism, which is brought on by the thyroid tissue's slow degradation. Assessing thyroid function and modifying medication dosage as necessary require routine blood test monitoring of thyroid hormone levels, including TSH, Free T4, and Free T3.

Goiter:

Sometimes, an enlargement of the thyroid gland can result in the formation of a goiter. Thyroid gland features and size can be monitored using routine physical examinations and, if needed, imaging procedures like ultrasonography.

Nodules on the Thyroid:

Thyroid nodules can arise in people with Hashimoto's thyroiditis. Even though the majority of nodules are benign, routine ultrasonography monitoring and, if necessary, a small needle aspiration biopsy can assist identify any nodules that need more assessment or care.

Immune System Disorders:

As an autoimmune disease, Hashimoto's thyroiditis may put a person at higher risk of getting other autoimmune diseases like type 1 diabetes or rheumatoid arthritis. It could be advised to have regular examinations and to watch for symptoms of further autoimmune illnesses.

Complications related to the heart:

Untreated hypothyroidism raises the risk of high blood pressure, heart disease, and high cholesterol, among other cardiovascular problems. It's crucial to regularly check cardiovascular health metrics and take care of any risk factors.

Mental Health Concerns:

Depression and cognitive decline are two mental health symptoms that can result from hypothyroidism. Comprehensive care includes monitoring mental health, getting help when needed, and dealing with any new problems.

Infertility and irregular menstruation:

Menstrual abnormalities and problems with conception might result from hypothyroidism linked to Hashimoto's thyroiditis. Planning to get pregnant can benefit from keeping an eye on and treating hormone abnormalities with the right treatments.

Obstetrical complications:

Hashimoto's thyroiditis patients may need extra care and modifications to their thyroid medication when they are pregnant. Pregnancy-related hypothyroidism that is not well managed or treated might put the developing fetus and the mother at danger.

Bone Well-being:

Osteoporosis and other bone-related disorders can result from hypothyroidism. It's crucial to keep an eye on bone density and take proactive steps to maintain bone health, such as getting enough calcium and vitamin D in your diet.

Frequent Follow-Up Meetings:

Patients with Hashimoto's thyroiditis should schedule routine follow-up visits with endocrinologists and other medical professionals. During these consultations, thyroid function may be evaluated via blood testing, physical examinations, and talks about general health and wellbeing.

Tailored Care:

Understand that the monitoring strategy is customized for each patient, and that the number of follow-up appointments and tests could change depending on the patient's reaction to therapy, the severity of their Hashimoto's thyroiditis, and the existence of comorbidities.

People with Hashimoto's Thyroiditis can effectively manage their illness and enhance general well-being by closely monitoring thyroid function, swiftly addressing any emergent issues, and using a complete approach to therapy. Maintaining regular contact with healthcare specialists guarantees that the management plan is in line with each patient's needs and objectives.

CONCLUSION

To sum up, Hashimoto's Thyroiditis is a complicated autoimmune condition that has a major influence on thyroid function and general health. The disorder, named for Dr. Hakaru Hashimoto, was initially reported in 1912. It is characterized by the immune system misfiring against the thyroid gland, causing inflammation, progressive thyroid tissue death, and hypothyroidism.

The path of Hashimoto's Thyroiditis involves several facets, from the first mild symptoms to the continuous thyroid function maintenance and possible problems. The following are important factors to take into account if you have Hashimoto's thyroiditis:

Nature of Autoimmune:

awareness Hashimoto's thyroiditis requires an awareness of its autoimmune nature. The thyroid gland is under attack by the immune system, which emphasizes how critical it is to treat both the autoimmune reaction and the ensuing hypothyroidism.

Living Style and Psychological Health:

Supporting general well-being requires incorporating lifestyle factors including stress management, frequent exercise, and a nutritious diet. A holistic approach to living with Hashimoto's thyroiditis must prioritize emotional well-being and cultivate a positive outlook.

Medical Care:

The mainstay of medical care is thyroid hormone replacement medication, usually with levothyroxine. Effective management involves adhering to recommended drug regimen consistently, routinely checking thyroid function by blood tests, and adjusting medication dosage.

Problems and Observation:

Knowing about possible side effects, like goiter, hypothyroidism, thyroid nodules, and related concerns, emphasizes how crucial routine monitoring is. Physical tests, imaging studies, and routine follow-up appointments can help identify changes and quickly address new problems.

Tailored Care:

Understanding that every person's experience with Hashimoto's thyroiditis is different highlights the importance of providing tailored treatment. The overall management of the condition is improved when treatment regimens, lifestyle modifications, and emotional support are customized to each individual's unique needs and objectives.

Knowledge and Self-determination:

People who are informed about Hashimoto's thyroiditis are better able to take an active role in their own care. Those who are well-informed about the illness, available treatments, and possible lifestyle factors are more equipped to make decisions and speak out for their own health.

In the end, treating Hashimoto's thyroiditis is a continuous process that calls for proactive communication and cooperation between patients and their medical professionals. People with Hashimoto's thyroiditis can maximize their health, reduce difficulties, and lead satisfying lives by treating the autoimmune component, controlling thyroid function, and adopting a holistic approach to well-being. A good outlook, self-care dedication, and regular communication all help people navigate the complexity of Hashimoto's thyroiditis with resilience and empowerment.

THE END